The information contained in this booklet is not intended as medical advice to the individual reader and is not a substitute for a consultation with your physician. Neither the author nor the publisher shall be liable or responsible for any loss, injury or damage allegedly arising from any suggestion or information contained in this booklet.

For more information or to contact the author, visit her website at:
www.SimpleHealthNetwork.com
or on Facebook at: Simple Health Network

The Real Story About Oxidation and Antioxidants
Copyright 2012 by Simple Health Network, Spokane, WA

Author Dr. Peggy Parker
Library of Congress Cataloging-in-Publication Data
Parker, Peggy, ND, Biological Medicine Diplomat
ISBN 978-0-9847997-4-9
Health - Medical
Printed in the United States of America,
First Printing October 2012

The Real Story About Oxidation & Antioxidants

by Dr. Peggy Parker

Everyday your body wages a silent war against elements of destruction that are so tiny they can only be seen by a powerful electron microscope, but their effects are as clear as the lines on your face . . .

- ✔ Their devestation is responsible for aging, disease and ultimately death . . .

- ✔ For decades doctors and medical researchers have studied them and have only found way to slow their progress . . .

Until now . . .

- ✔ Now a cutting edge technology provides the ultimate solution to anti-aging and disease prevention . . .

- ✔ It allows you to stop free radicals in their tracks . . .

- ✔ Since all antioxidants are NOT the same you deserve to know . . .

The Real Story About Oxidation and Antioxidants

You've read the articles, seen the news clips, and even watched the movies outlining the hazards chemical spills, dangerous nuclear melt down and chemical additives to our food and water have on our health.

Each of these dangerous incidents had a dramatic impact on the lives of every person living nearby.

But you may not realize that there is an even more deadly silent killer that attacks you each and every day. Its effects have been studied countless times by tens of thousands of medical researchers . . .

Oxidation caused by free radicals is the culprit behind aging, disease and death.

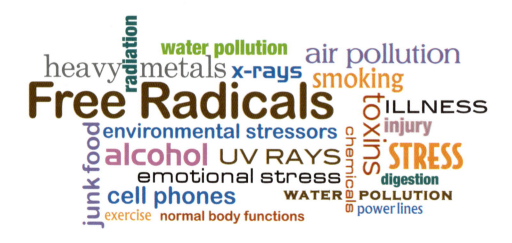

It seems our modern lifestyle has escalated free radical devastation to epidemic proportions . . .

Not a day goes by that you don't see another article or hear another news report announcing the connection between these silent killers and yet another health hazard.

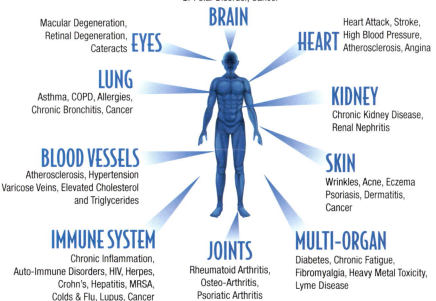

Leaving doctors, scientists and medical researchers asking themselves . . .

How Can We Stop Them?

Scientists, medical researchers and biologists have performed tens of thousands of research studies on foods and vitamins and antioxidants.

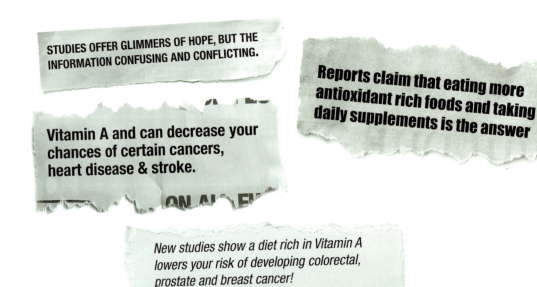

But then other reports surface with headlines like:

These potential problems are not limited to Vitamin A – it includes all antioxidants – A, C and E!

Research has demonstrated that while the antioxidants we find in food and even supplements offer some benefits, there are also some surprising downsides. Here are a few things you should know . . .

- ✔ Only about 25% of the antioxidants in food and supplements can be utilized by your body . . . this is the result of both poor digestion and oxidized cell membranes.
- ✔ In high doses certain antioxidants can become toxic to the liver . . . fat soluble vitamins like Vitamins A and E can build up in your tissues and have some serious consequences to your health.
- ✔ As antioxidants do their job they add to the burden of free radicals in your body.
- ✔ Antioxidants are tissue specific . . . each antioxidant is only effectively used by certain cells or tissues.

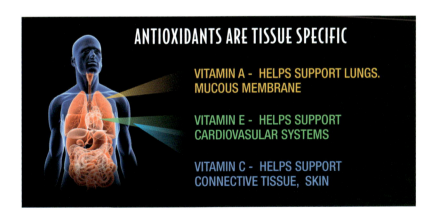

In other words, antioxidants are not universally available to stop the destructive cycle of oxidation.

BUT...

what if there was ONE very special antioxidant that had the power to reverse all of these health conditions . . .

And wouldn't it be great if it was easy to get, inexpensive and could neutralize ALL free radicals everywhere in the body . . .

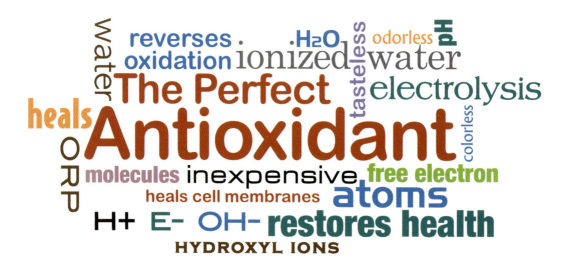

Wouldn't you want that antioxidant?

Dr. Peggy Parker made a ground-breaking medical discovery . . .

She uncovered the real story of oxidation and the single most effective antioxidant available today. . .

Until now, no one understood it . . .

No one knew this simple antioxidant has the power to stop oxidation at its source . . .

It has been completely overlooked or misunderstood by medical researchers, scientists and physicians . . .

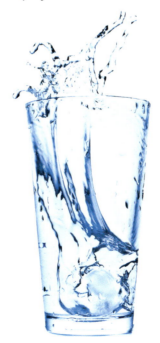

And you can find it in a glass of water . . .

The story starts with your cells.

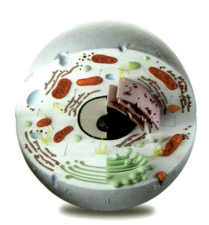

Your body is composed of 70-100 trillion cells which all have a few things in common?

Each of these cells is surrounded by a cell membrane made primarily of fat, called a phospholipid bilayer.

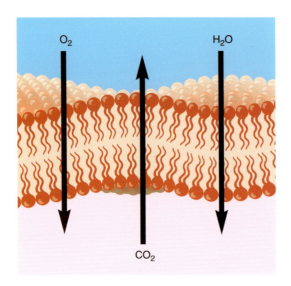

A healthy cell membrane is selectively permeable. It allows water and oxygen to flow freely into the cell.

This keeps it properly hydrated, pH balanced and ready to produce energy. It also allows carbon dioxide and other waste products to flow freely out of the cell.

Special proteins are imbedded into the cell membrane that regulate the transfer of minerals, hormones, vitamins, enzymes and other nutrients into and out of the cell.

This process is referred to as cellular transport.

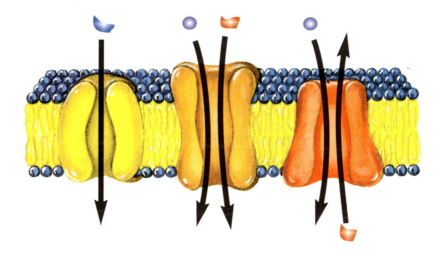

Did you know . . . that the overall health of your body is determined by the health of the cell membrane?

You see, healthy cell membranes create healthy cells, and healthy cells make healthy tissues, and healthy tissues make healthy bodies.

But . . .
we have one major problem!

Every day, each of those 70-100 trillion cells that make up your body is assaulted 10,000 times by damaging free radicals!

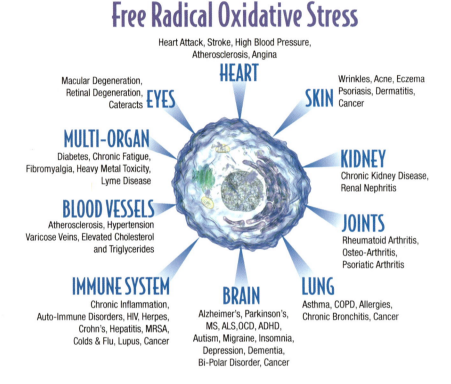

As you can see, the cellular damage created by these free radicals affects every part of your body.

Oxidative damage is such a widespread problem that it has been linked to virtually every illness or disease, as shown in countless studies, performed by thousands of doctors and medical researchers.

The one thing they all agree on is that over time these elements of destruction begin to damage otherwise healthy organs, tissues, and cells down to your DNA.

As these free radicals attack the weak links in your genetic chain, they can damage your DNA and leave you at a much greater risk for illness, disease and even premature death, but . . .

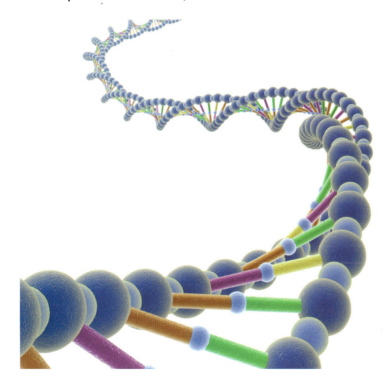

. . . *your DNA is not your destiny!*

Despite tens of thousands of scientific articles that verify the role of oxidation as the primary cause of aging and disease, no one really understood the process . . . *that is until now!*

After many years of clinical research, Dr. Peggy Parker connected the dots . . . She outlined the downward cycle of oxidation that leads to disease and aging.

The cycle begins when healthy cell membranes become damaged by free radical oxidation. As the damage from oxidation progresses the cell membrane actually changes.

The oxidized fats in the cell membrane are no longer fluid, flexible and permeable but instead become thick, sticky and impermeable . . .

Just like the oxidized fat on your kitchen exhaust fan!

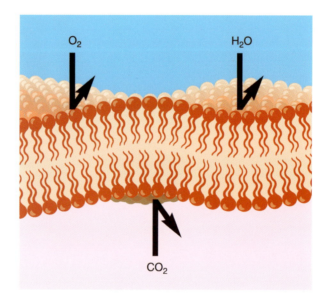

The thick, sticky fats in the cell membrane are no longer able to allow the free passage of water and oxygen into the cell, or the carbon dioxide and other waste products out of the cell.

As cells become burdened with toxic wastes and even more free radicals, a greater imbalance in the natural pH occurs, until these cells become hopelessly dehydrated.

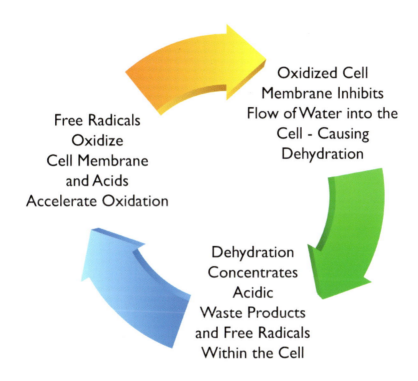

This accumulation of acids, waste products and free radicals leads to further oxidation of the cell membrane, and so the downward cycle of oxidation continues.

Now that you understand the gravity of the situation, here's how it happened . . .

Let's start with the basics . . .

Atoms are the building blocks of your cells, and all stable atoms contain an even number of paired electrons.

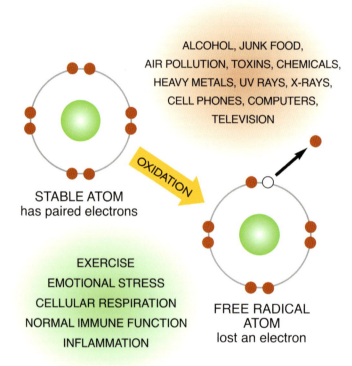

Free radicals occur when stable atoms lose an electron, resulting in a single, unstable, unpaired electron.

Many things in our surroundings, including the UV rays emitted by the sun, radiation from our cell phones, computers and televisions, and even the food we eat, create these unstable free radicals. Surprisingly enough, so do many natural functions in our bodies. Exercise and even emotional stress are also part of the problem!

In fact, your cells are free radical producing factories! As cells produce energy, they burn oxygen, leaving behind - you guessed it - free radicals! As your immune system kills foreign invaders, it actually uses free radicals!

The end result is that all of these things contribute to the production of destructive free radicals!

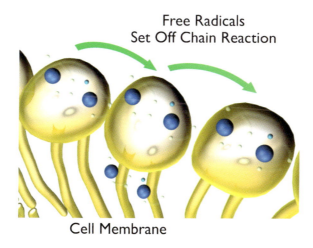

Free Radicals Set Off Chain Reaction

Cell Membrane

Once created, these free radicals set off a chain reaction that begins a never ending cycle of oxidative damage, aging, disease and ultimately, death. And it all begins with your cell membrane!

Now here's the good news . . .

Dr. Parker made a groundbreaking, scientific discovery that changes everything! She uncovered the surprisingly simple solution to the incredibly complex subject of oxidation.

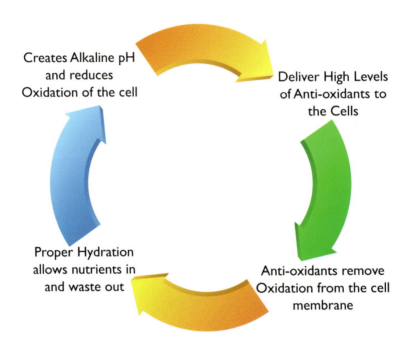

She discovered the cycle of oxidation can be reversed by delivering high levels of antioxidants to the cells. These antioxidants restore the cell membrane back to health. Healthy cell membranes once again allow oxygen and water to flow freely into the cell and wastes out of the cell.

This re-activates the body's self-healing cycle!

Now that you understand the benefits of antioxidants, here's how they work . . .

To stop the downward cycle of oxidation, the free radical must become stable again. That single, unpaired electron must find a mate!

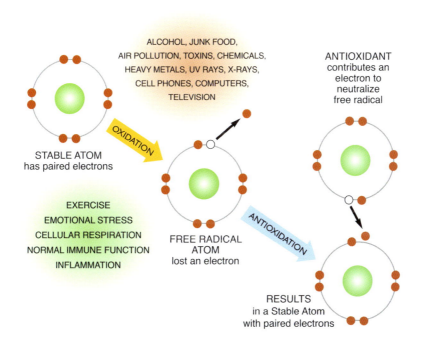

Antioxidants have the unique ability to donate an electron, transforming the free radical back into a stable atom!

While they are clearly beneficial, not all antioxidants are created equal . . .

Despite their obvious importance, antioxidants all suffer from one significant drawback you can clearly see . . .

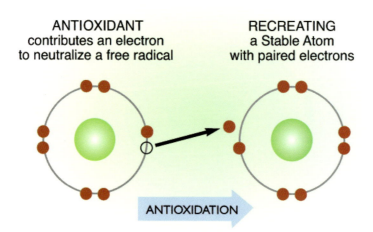

. . . by donating an electron to neutralize a free radical, the antioxidant now becomes a new free radical!

In other words, they actually add yet another free radical to the never ending cycle of oxidation, illness, disease and death!

Now to be perfectly clear, the antioxidant DID neutralize a very destructive free radical, and in exchange became a much weaker free radical. So while they do slow down the path to aging, disease and death . . . the downward spiral still continues!

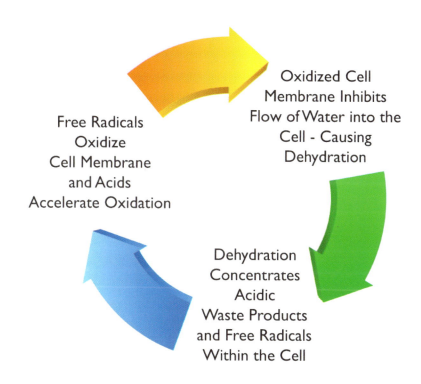

This problem left even the most brilliant scientists, doctors and researchers baffled, asking this question . . .

How can we stop this cycle of oxidation?

The solution to this perplexing problem turned out to be as simple as drinking a glass of water!

But not just any water . . . high quality ionized water!

The remarkable antioxidant properties of this water have been observed by many, but never understood . . . yet the principles are used by scientists, chemists and engineers every day.

High Quality Ionized Water

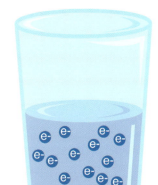

You see, high quality ionized water is rich in the most elegantly simple antioxidant that can be found . . . the free electron.

Creating free electrons is nothing new. In fact a high quality water ionizer treats water the same way a hydrogen fuel cell does.

And it happens like this . . .

When an electrical current passes through water, a process known as electrolysis, some of the water molecules break apart, creating Hydroxyl Ions (OH-) and Hydrogen Gas (H).

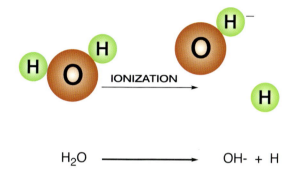

$H_2O \longrightarrow$ OH- + H

And just like in a hydrogen fuel cell, when the Hydrogen molecules are exposed to platinum, they release their electrons!

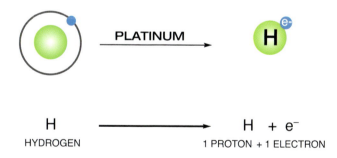

H $\longrightarrow$ H + e⁻
HYDROGEN   1 PROTON + 1 ELECTRON

In a hydrogen fuel cell, these electrons are directed down a wire where they produce electricity.

But in a high quality water ionizer, these free electrons become part of the alkaline drinking water.

One of the most important things to keep in mind in the process of creating free electrons through ionization is this . . . the stronger the electrical current passing through the water, the more hydrogen gas is produced . . .

And the more platinum the hydrogen gas is exposed to, the greater the number of free electrons produced.

And those free electrons are just that . . . **FREE!**

RECREATING
a Stable Atom
with a Free Electron

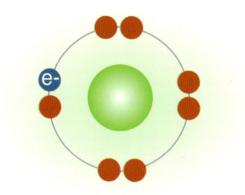

Free to neutralize any free radical anywhere in your body!